❧ *LISINOPRIL* ☙

Excellent Guide to Treat High Blood Pressure (Hypertension), Diabetes Affecting Eyes & Kidneys; Prevent Heart Attack or Failure & be Side Effect-Free

Dr. Lovel Martins

Table of Contents

Introduction

Angiotensin Converting Enzyme inhibitors (medications that help relax the veins and arteries to lower blood pressure), such as Lisinopril, are oral long-acting medications. It is a lysine-derived form of Enalprilate and resembles its precursor structurally. The absence of the Sulfhydryl group makes it different from Captopril.

Lisinopril is used to treat hypertension, congestive heart failure, heart attacks, as well as diabetic problems involving the kidneys and eyes.

Additionally, it shows haemodynamic effects. It is an inhibitor with active site specificity. It encourages natriuresis and aids type II diabetic patients in avoiding diabetic retinopathy.

Both angiotensin-converting enzyme inhibitors and angiotensin receptor blockers are equally advised as first-line treatments for hypertension since they both successfully decrease blood pressure by inhibiting the renin-angiotensin pathway.

Angiotensin Converting Enzyme Inhibitors are strongly advised as first-line agents for the start of antihypertensive therapy based on the highest level of evidence in both the 2017 American College of Cardiology/American Heart Association and the 2018 European Society of Cardiology/European Society of Hypertension guidelines on hypertension.

It starts working after one to two hours. Action lasts for 24 hours. Lisinopril is absorbed from the mouth slowly and moderately, reaching its peak plasma concentration after 7 hours.

It interacts with some medications but it does not interact with meals. Up to 25% of drugs are distributed. It does not go through a metabolic process and is eliminated unaltered in urine. When hypertension is present, the medication is taken orally.

The first adult dosage is 5-10 mg daily administered before night. 2.5-5 mg of medication once daily is the starting dose for renovascular hypertension, volume depletion, and severe hypertension. 5 mg once daily in individuals on diuretics up to 80 mg of the maintenance dosage may be administered.

There is extensive evidence that blood pressure lowering by renin-angiotensin system inhibition using Lisinopril drug improves cardiovascular outcomes

In this book, I will extensively discuss, the secret of Lisinopril, its working principles, its side effects, precautions, benefits and as well as warnings for pregnant and breastfeeding mothers.

Also, all the basis of Hypertension, how Lisinopril combats hypertension, complications of hypertension, those who are at risk of having hypertension and as well as the causes of hypertension will be discussed in this book.

I am very sure you will enjoy every bit of this book especially if you are tired of your problems and you no longer know how to scale through.

I will walk you through how you will take Lisinopril without experiencing any complications. And I will ensure the entire secret you do not know about Lisinopril and how it treats hypertension is clearly exposed.

Chapter One

Understanding Lisinopril Medication

Lisinopril is an oral medication and angiotensin converting enzyme inhibitors. It is used to treat and successfully prevent Hypertension (high blood pressure) in both children and adults. This drug should not be administered to children under the age of six.

When a heart attack happens, some of the heart muscle can be weakened and damaged. Lisinopril is used to treat previously survived heart attacks in patients with cardiac abnormalities and can also be used to treat adult heart failure.

With the usage of Lisinopril, the process of reducing blood pressure reduces the risk of deadly and non-fatal cardiovascular effects such as strokes, renal issues, and heart attacks.

Additionally, this drug can be used to successfully lessen heart attack and heart failure symptoms, especially in adults.

When given within 24 hours of a myocardial infarction or heart failure that may develop without warning, Lisinopril can also increase survival.

For the treatment of hypertension, this medicine may be used either on its own or in conjunction with other medications.

This drug works by preventing the substances in the body system that cause blood vessels to constrict, which in turn causes the arteries, veins, and capillaries to relax. This lowers blood pressure and increases blood flow to the heart area.

If hypertension (high blood pressure) is not properly controlled, it can harm the kidneys, brain, heart, blood vessels, and other organs.

Heart disease, a heart attack, heart failure, a stroke, renal failure, eyesight loss, and other issues may develop from damage to these organs.

More specifically, taking medicine and altering your lifestyle will both reduce your blood pressure. These adjustments include quitting smoking, drinking alcohol in moderation, eating a diet low in fat and salt, keeping a healthy weight, and exercising for at least 30 minutes every day. Lisinopril reduces blood volume, which in turn lowers blood pressure by inhibiting chemical reactions that help the body retain water and salt.

For the treatment of hypertension, Lisinopril combines two medications that can be administered alongside calcium channel blockers and diuretics.

The Features of Lisinopril

Lisinopril comes in the form of a white, crystalline powder with a molar mass of 40.488 g/mol and a molecular weight of 441.52.

Lisinopril has a molecular weight of 441.53 and is available as a white to off-white, crystalline powder. It is essentially insoluble in ethanol, acetone, acetonitrile, and chloroform, and sparingly soluble in methanol and water.

How Lisinopril Works?

Lisinopril works by blocking the conversion of angiotensin I to angiotensin II, a strong vasoconstrictor, by acting as a competitive inhibitor of the angiotensin-converting enzyme. With the usage of Lisinopril, a minor rise in serum potassium may occur because a drop in angiotensin II leads to a decrease in aldosterone (a hormone that increases sodium absorption by the kidneys, controlling the equilibrium of salt and water) secretion, which in turn causes a decrease in sodium reabsorption in the collecting duct and a decrease in potassium excretion.

Lisinopril causes an increase in serum renin activity by eliminating the angiotensin II's negative feedback mechanism.

The favorable benefits in hypertension patients come from the renin-angiotensin-aldosterone system's inhibitory actions, which lead to lower aldosterone activity even in patients with low renin levels.

However, Angiotensin Converting Enzyme also breaks down bradykinin, and it is because of this mechanism that Angiotensin Converting Enzyme inhibitors may increase the risk of angioedema.

This process makes it easy for Lisinopril to relax the arteries, and decrease how hard the heart has to work to pump blood throughout the body to reduce blood pressure.

Chapter Two

Understanding Hypertension (High Blood Pressure)

Blood pressure is the amount of pressure that blood applies to the walls of blood vessels in order to transport blood through them. The heart also pushes blood against the walls of the arteries as it pumps it throughout the body.

Blood pressure is influenced by the distance between the heart and the arteries, capillaries, and veins that carry blood. The blood arteries around the heart show signs of high blood pressure. This shows that the blood pressure in the arterial circulation is higher than in the venous circulation.

13

This occurs as a result of the thick artery walls, which force the artery walls to contract, being less flexible than the vein walls, which are thin and have more elasticity.

Numerous factors can affect someone's blood pressure. These factors include the amount of blood in the body, how hard the heart has to work, the kind of blood, how flexible the blood arteries are, and the permeability of the blood.

High blood pressure is a common condition in the US that increases the risk of coronary heart disease and stroke. Blood pushing against the walls of arteries in the body causes pressure, which frequently varies during the day.

High blood pressure, often known as hypertension, is when it is regularly higher than what is regarded as normal.

There are blood pressure readings for both the systolic and diastolic states. Diastolic blood pressure describes the force on the arteries at rest, whereas systolic blood pressure describes the force on the arteries during beating.

Less than 120/80 mm Hg, or less than 80 mm Hg for the diastolic and less than 120 mm Hg for the systolic, is considered to be a good blood pressure measurement. Doctors may have somewhat varying definitions of high blood pressure since some guidelines state that it must consistently be more than 130/80 mm Hg while others state that it must be greater than 140/90 mm Hg.

If your blood pressure is excessively high, it puts additional strain on your heart and blood vessels. If left untreated or unnoticed, this added strain over time may cause organ damage, increasing your risk of developing health problems.

If you have high blood pressure and don't control it, your risk of having a heart attack or stroke rises. High blood pressure can damage your arteries; result in heart disease, renal disease, and eye problems. It is also a risk factor for some kinds of vascular dementia.

What Kinds of Hypertension Exist?

Depending on how severe it is, hypertension falls into a variety of groups. Hypertension comes in two main forms. These varieties include **Essential Hypertension** also known as primary hypertension and **Non-Essential Hypertension** also known as secondary hypertension. Let's get into further depth about these two.

Essential Hypertension

When peripheral resistance is increasing the blood pressure in the arteries, essential hypertension develops.

In cases of essential hypertension, arterial pressure increases by 50%, and renal blood flow eventually decreases. Additionally, the barrier to blood flow via the kidney increases 2-4 times. Until the artery's pressure is raised, the kidney will not expel adequate salt and water.

Other forms of essential hypertension exist. These include:

Malignant Hypertension:

In this type of hypertension, the systolic and diastolic blood pressures are elevated to between 240 and 250 mmHg and 140 and 150 mmHg, respectively. Serious health issues include ocular illness, renal disease, kidney disease, as well as mortality, might be caused by malignant hypertension.

Benign Hypertension:

This is characterized by an increase in blood pressure with a systolic pressure of around 200 mmHg and a diastolic pressure of approximately 100 mmHg.

However, if there is adequate rest and relaxation, the pressure could go back to normal.

What Causes Essential Hypertension?

The following are several frequent distinct variables that contribute to essential hypertension:

- Lack of exercise and inactivity.
- Obesity/overweight.
- Insulin resistance.

- Renin-angiotension system.
- Sympathetic nervous system.
- Genetic component.
- Increase salt intake.
- Nutrition throughout pregnancy and low birth weight.

Non-essential Hypertension

Different kinds of non-essential hypertension exist. These consist of:

Endocrine hypertension:

This condition is brought on by excess cortisone secretion, tumors in the adrenal medulla, excess growth hormone secretion, and excess aldosterone secretion from the adrenal cortex (Conn's syndrome).

Renal hypertension:

This condition results from the constriction of one or both renal arteries, which impairs renal function and causes nephron or renal glomeruli inflammation.

Cardiovascular hypertension:

This condition is brought on by the aorta narrowing and the blood vessels hardening and narrowing (atherosclerosis).

Causes of Non-essential Hypertension

Secondary hypertension is caused by a variety of reasons. Among these elements are:

Renal Contributors

Example of a renal etiology of secondary hypertension

- Renal artery stenosis
- Diabetic kidney disease
- Polycystic kidney disease
- Glomerulonephritis.

Endocrine contributors

Examples of endocrine etiology of non-essential hypertension includes:

- Acromegaly.
- Exogenous hormones,
- Phaeochromocytoma.

- Hypothyroidism.

- Cushing's syndrome.

- Conn's syndrome.

- Hyperparathyroidism.

Additional contributors

Some examples are:

i.   Hypertension associated with pregnancy.

ii.   Coarctation of the aorta.

iii.   Acute stress

iv.   Alcohol.

Effects of High Blood Pressure

Long-term or persistently high blood pressure may cause damage to the arterial walls. The artery might also be strained, which could result in a number of problems.

Hypertension can affect some organs. This occurs in the following techniques:

The artery's capacity to transport blood is firstly blocked. Coronary artery disease, peripheral arterial disease, and stroke are all conditions brought on by atherosclerosis (blocked artery).

Next, the arteries begin to rupture. Aortic valve dissection and cerebral hemorrhage are the effects of this.

Another adverse effect of hypertension is that the medicines used to treat it might affect different organs (anti-hypertensive drugs). This might create a couple of more problems. These include:

- Disease of the peripheral arteries.
- Retinopathy.
- Heart disease.
- Kidney failure brought on by trauma.
- Metabolic Syndrome.
- Aneurysm.
- Vision loss.
- Memory difficulties.
- Impotence issues.
- Left ventricular hypertrophy and failure.
- Dementia.
- Atrioventricular fibrillation.

- Cardiac attack.

High Blood Pressure Symptoms

Hypertension frequently goes undetected and without signs. Without a diagnosis, you won't be able to say for sure if you have hypertension.

There are a few signs you may look out for to see if you have hypertension or not, but not all symptoms suggest that you have; a test is the only way to know for sure.

Examples of these indications include:

- Heartbeats, ear beats, and maybe other area in the body.
- Breathing difficulties
- Neck ache in the back.
- Dizziness.
- The pulse or beat is out of balance.
- Drowsiness.
- Blood discovered in the urine.
- Fatigue.
- Nausea.
- Aches in the chest.

22

- Experiencing heat and flushing.

- Poor sleeping and seeing abilities.

- Prolonged episodes of severe headaches.

- Vomiting.

- Confusion.

Testing your Blood Pressure

Using a standard and verified blood pressure monitor, calibrated aneroid manometer, or a certified electronic device connected to the left arm should provide reliable blood pressure readings.

These steps are used to test blood pressure:

Systolic blood pressure is typically 90-119 mmHg, while diastolic blood pressure is 60-79 mmHg.

Blood pressure associated with pre-hypertension ranges from 120 to 139 mmHg systolic and 80 to 89 mmHg diastolic.

Measurements of stage 1 hypertension range from 140 to 159 mmHg systolic and 90 to 99 mmHg diastolic.

The systolic and diastolic pressures for stage 2 hypertension are more than or equivalent to 160 and 100 mmHg, respectively.

Greater than or equal to 140 mmHg systolic and less than 90 mmHg diastolic pressures are indicators of isolated systolic hypertension.

Chapter Three

Understanding Congestive Heart Failure

Congestive heart failure mostly affects the elderly, occurring in up to 10% of those over the age of 80, and its frequency is growing.

Heart failure is a condition in which the heart is unable to produce enough cardiac output to satisfy the body's metabolic needs and allow for venous return. Dyspnea, orthopnea, and weariness are among the symptoms that contribute to the diagnosis, along with indicators like pulmonary and peripheral oedema.

Heart damage with the loss or impairment of functional myocardial cells is the end consequence of a variety of distinct pathophysiological processes.

Heart rate and cardiac smooth muscle contraction are increased by sympathetic nervous system activation, but salt absorption and water retention are increased by renin-angiotensin-aldosterone system activity.

Despite the fact that these reactions are initially advantageous, sustained overstimulation of the sympathetic nervous system and the renin-angiotensin-aldosterone system leads to maladaptive cardiovascular remodeling.

The sympathetic nervous system's and the renin-angiotensin-aldosterone system's vasoconstrictions actions are countered by the release of natriuretic peptides.

What may Happen when you have Congestive Heart Failure?

- *Your heart is not pumping blood effectively enough.*

- *Your veins clog up with blood.*
- *As fluid accumulates throughout your body, your feet, ankles, and legs may become swollen. We refer to this as "edema."*
- *Your lungs fill with fluid. We refer to this as "pulmonary edema."*
- *Your body doesn't receive enough oxygen, food, or blood.*

Ejection Rate (Fraction)

Myocardial dysfunction is a common cause of heart failure, which is widely categorized by left ventricular ejection fraction. Heart failure with decreased ejection fraction is characterized by a left ventricular ejection fraction of less than 40%.

Heart failure with intact ejection fraction is the medical term for a situation when the ejection fraction is at least 50%. About 50% of all heart failure cases are caused by this.

Although the presentation and heart failure with decreased ejection fraction are clinically identical, the two conditions require distinct treatments.

The European Society of Cardiology recently defined "mid-range" left ventricular ejection fraction as being between 40 and 49%. However, this is a complex subject that needs additional investigation due to the variability in determining left ventricular ejection percent.

Angiotensin Receptor Antagonists and Angiotensin Converting Enzyme Inhibitors

First-line treatment for heart failure with low ejection fraction and asymptomatic left ventricular dysfunction is angiotensin-converting enzyme inhibitors.

With a decrease in myocardial infarction and heart failure hospitalization, its usage resulted in a 3.8% absolute reduction (20% relative) in mortality.

In all age groups, beneficial benefits start early and last a long time. Adenosine and water retention, vasoconstriction, and heart hypertrophy and fibrosis are all maladaptive outcomes of prolonged renin-angiotensin-aldosterone system activation that are lessened by angiotensin-converting enzyme inhibitors.

Symptoms of Congestive Heart Failure

- Weight increase due to fluid retention.
- Dizziness or difficulty thinking clearly.
- Feeling faint or dizzy.
- Breathing difficulties, especially while resting down.
- Feeling drained and worn-out (fatigue).
- Coughing or wheezing, particularly after exercising or when lying down.
- Legs, ankles, and foot swelling.

Causes of Congestive Heart Failure

High blood pressure and Coronary Artery Disease are the two most frequent causes of heart failure in the United States.

Coronary Artery Disease develops when plaque buildups in the arteries that carry blood to the heart muscle cause them to constrict.

Other typical risk factors for heart failure include:

29

- High triglycerides.
- Hyperglycemia syndrome.
- Sleep apnea.
- Abuse of drugs or alcohol.
- Having a weight problem.
- Type 2 Diabetes.
- Cigarettes.

The following conditions can also result in cardiac failure:

- An abnormal cardiac rhythm.
- Infection of the heart and/or heart valves (arrhythmias).
- A previous cardiac attack that left the heart muscle somewhat damaged.
- Birth malformations in the heart.
- Disease of the heart valves.
- Heart muscle disorders.

Smoking and Lisinopril Usage

It is well recognized that elevated blood pressure, or hypertension, is the main factor in human cardiovascular illnesses. The primary ingredient in cigarettes, nicotine, enters the bloodstream as soon as a patient starts smoking. The consumption of nicotine may cause the arterioles to close, raising blood pressure as a result.

Most smokers frequently suffer blood flow obstruction and even chilly hands. Because the heart must pump blood to the lungs, particularly when there is a decline in the capacity to carry oxygen, this can be quite serious.

In patients on angiotensin converting enzyme inhibitor therapy (Lisinopril), smoking may be a recognized risk factor for the advancement of chronic renal disease associated with primary hypertension.

Combining Lisinopril with Alcohol

It is important to be aware of any potential interactions, negative side effects, and risks while combining Lisinopril with alcohol.

First off, combining Lisinopril with alcohol might make the medication less effective.

Studies on the interaction between alcohol and Lisinopril have revealed that excessive alcohol consumption is a common cause of high blood pressure and can worsen the issues that the medication is intended to alleviate. Low blood pressure is a potential side effect of alcohol with Lisinopril.

When you consume alcohol while taking Lisinopril, your blood pressure may occasionally decrease to the point that you feel symptoms like lightheadedness.

Fainting or other significant adverse effects might result from having too low of blood pressure. Dizziness can be a side effect of alcohol or Lisinopril taken alone, as well as the combination of the two; as a result, drinking alcohol while taking Lisinopril may make these symptoms worse. Avoid taking Lisinopril with alcohol if you've found that it causes you to feel dizzy even without it.

Drinking alcohol is never a good idea, and this is especially true if you're using Lisinopril, since the side effects of both medications might be worsened when combined.

Given the impact alcohol can have on your blood pressure, including the ability to cause it to drop too low or rise too high, it is not recommended that you combine alcohol with Lisinopril for any reason.

When you combine alcohol with Lisinopril, there is also a danger of increased dizziness and a risk of fainting.

In the end, you should always discuss your health history with your doctors, as well as any potential interactions, side effects, and risks of consuming alcohol while taking Lisinopril. You should also constantly be aware of how you respond to the medication.

Lisinopril Uses and Benefits

The following are some of the factors that make Lisinopril a very successful drug for treating hypertension.

Heart failure, heart attacks, and high blood pressure are among conditions that are treated with Lisinopril.

With the usage of Lisinopril, the process of reducing blood pressure reduces the risk of deadly and non-fatal cardiovascular effects such as strokes, renal issues, and heart attacks.

Lisinopril is used to treat adult heart failure as well as heart failure in patients who have already survived a heart attack (after a heart attack, some heart muscle might be damaged and weakened). Patients with heart anomalies may also use this medication to treat other heart conditions.

When given within 24 hours of a myocardial infarction or heart failure that may develop without warning, Lisinopril can also increase survival.

Additionally, this drug can be used to successfully lessen heart attack and heart failure symptoms, especially in adults.

This drug is used to treat and prevent hypertension (high blood pressure) in both adults and children. This drug should not be administered to children under the age of six.

Chapter Four

Lisinopril with Low Blood Pressure (Hypotension)

Hypotension, a condition marked by low blood pressure, may occur within the first few days of starting this medication's use. You can notice signs and symptoms which include headaches, lightheadedness, dizziness, and fainting. Don't hesitate to call your doctor right away.

If you see any of the following, hypotension can start to develop:

- If you don't drink enough water.
- If you suffer from heart failure.
- In case you use diuretics (water pills).

- If you're perspiring a lot.
- In the event that you have renal dialysis.
- If you're constipated.
- If you're throwing up.

Methods for Using Lisinopril

Before using this medication, please carefully read the directions on the product package.

A glass of water must be consumed when taking Lisinopril.

To ensure that you are not given an under dose or an overdose of this drug, the dosage instructions must be precisely followed.

Although you can take this medication with or without food, it is best to do so after eating.

For optimal monitoring, this drug must be taken exactly as prescribed by doctors or physicians.

Make careful to regularly check your blood pressure, especially when using this medicine.

If you experience any of these side effects while taking this medication, contact your doctor right away. Dehydration can also cause low blood pressure, kidney problems, and electrolyte imbalances.

Surgery may be necessary for some patients depending on their condition. Before beginning to take Lisinopril, be sure to inform your doctor.

Because high blood pressure can occasionally be asymptomatic, patients who are taking this medicine for the treatment of high blood pressure should keep doing so even if they no longer exhibit the symptoms. Therefore, you must continue taking this drug for a long period or for the rest of your life.

The dosage of this drug depends on the medical condition you are treating and how you react to it.

Children's dosages for this drug are determined by weight. A youngster who is underweight receives a lower dosage than a child who is healthy weight.

While people using it to treat heart failure may need to take it for more than 4 weeks to see results, those taking it to treat high blood pressure often get improvement within 2-4 weeks of starting therapy.

Doctors might suggest that you begin taking this medicine at a lesser dose and gradually increase it. To lessen the possibility of serious adverse effects, this is done.

In order to have the best results, this medicine dose regimen must be followed exactly as prescribed by the doctor. You must take this medicine exactly as prescribed if it is prescribed to be taken every 24 hours.

Lisinopril Caution

The guidelines stated below should be properly followed by the following group of patients who have various medical issues.

Patients with Diabetes: Lisinopril usage when you have diabetes may impact your blood sugar level. If you need to adjust your diabetic medication dosage or reduce how much you take it, call your doctor right away.

Patients with Dysfunctional Kidneys: Lisinopril usage may impair renal function in patients with dysfunctional kidneys. Before recommending this drug to you, make sure your doctor is aware of any renal issues you may have.

People who suffer Elevated Potassium Levels: Lisinopril usage may increase or enhance your body's potassium levels, which may then cause a serious heart rate problem. This rise in potassium level might occasionally take place quickly.

Patients with Heart Issues: If you have a condition called hypertrophic cardiomyopathy or stenosis, using this medicine may lower your blood pressure.

Patients who suffer from a Chronic Cough: Taking Lisinopril may worsen an existing persistent cough, which may then go away once you stop taking Lisinopril.

Precautions for Taking Lisinopril

To be sure the drug is truly helping you, ask your doctor to check on the progress of your recovery at each appointment. For the best medical outcome, further monitoring may be performed on you.

The use of this drug during pregnancy has the potential to damage or kill your unborn child. Make careful to stop using Lisinopril if you get pregnant, or use birth control pills to avoid becoming pregnant while taking this drug.

You should contact your doctor as soon as you notice any of these symptoms since using this drug can cause allergic responses including anaphylaxis, rash, itching, trouble breathing, hoarseness, difficulty swallowing, and swellings throughout the body.

While taking this medication, stomach pain is possible. The body may experience intestinal angioedema as a result of this. Get in touch with your doctor right away.

Getting up from a lying or sitting position or after taking a diuretic drug are the two main reasons why you might feel dizzy, lightheaded, or faint. Before driving, operating machinery, or engaging in other activities that could be hazardous if you are dizzy or inattentive, be sure to understand how the medication affects you.

To avoid passing out if you feel lightheaded, lie down. To avoid experiencing dizziness again, sit for a few seconds before standing.

If you notice that you are unwell while taking this medicine, make sure to call your doctor right away. You might get sick, throw up, and have diarrhea. As a result of this treatment, you may get dehydrated or lose too much salt, so be sure to drink enough of water.

While using Lisinopril, if you get a fever, chills, or sore throat, realize that this is an infection brought on by a lack of white blood cells in the body.

Do not take additional drugs unless your doctor has been informed. This includes over-the-counter (nonprescription) medications for regulating appetite, managing asthma, treating colds, cough, hay fever, or treating nasal issues since they have a tendency to raise blood pressure.

During the course of using this drug, a high amount of potassium may develop in the blood. The following symptoms might emerge as a result: nausea or vomiting, anxiety, numbness or tingling in the hands, feet, or lips, shortness of breath, weakness or heaviness in the legs, disorientation, breathing difficulties, irregular heartbeat, and abdominal or stomach discomfort. Make sure you consult your doctor before making any decisions.

Make sure to consult a doctor if you experience upper stomach pain, light-colored feces, dark urine, nausea, extreme fatigue or weakness, or yellow eyes or skin. These might be the outcome of a serious liver condition.

In black people, Lisinopril can be less effective. Angioedema is also more common in black people.

While taking this medicine, call your doctor right away if you see any signs of a high blood sugar level since Lisinopril may influence blood sugar levels.

Make sure your doctor is aware of your usage of Lisinopril since you might need to stop taking it a few days before having surgery.

Drug Interactions with Lisinopril

Drug interactions happen when one medicine you're taking affects how another one functions. This might be dangerous or make the other medication useless.

The following drugs may interact with Lisinopril:

Medication for High Blood Pressure

Lisinopril can result in low blood pressure, renal problems, kidney failure, and high blood potassium when used concurrently with other blood pressure drugs. These drugs include: Benazepril, Captopril, Enalapril, Fosinopril, Lisinopril, Moexipril, Candesartan, Eprosartan, Irbesartan, Losartan, and a number of other drugs are examples of this type of medication.

Low Blood Sugar Drugs

Taking Lisinopril with diabetic medications at the same time can significantly lower blood sugar levels. Insulin and diabetic oral medicines are two examples of such drugs.

Potassium Supplements

Combining Lisinopril with a potassium supplement may result in an elevated potassium level in the body. Examples of such drugs include: triamterene, amiloride, and spironolactone.

Diuretics

Hypotension (low blood pressure) may develop from concurrent use of diuretics and Lisinopril. Examples of such medications include:

- Hydrochlorothiazide.

- Furosemide.

- Bumetanide.

- Chlorthalidone.

Medication for Pain Relief

Combining Lisinopril with non-steroidal anti-inflammatory medicines may result in decreased renal function. These include:

- Diclofenac.

- Naproxen.

- Indomethacin.

- Ibuprofen.

- Flurbiprofen.

- Neprilysin inhibitors.

- Ketorolac.

- Sulindac.

- Aspirin.

- Ketoprofen.

If you have low blood salt levels, your doctor may recommend starting you on 2.5 mg of Lisinopril once daily.

For the first three days following a heart attack, your initial dose may be 2.5 mg if you have low blood pressure.

Tips and Advice about Lisinopril

One comprehensive cardiovascular risk reduction strategy that can target diabetes risk reduction, cholesterol reduction, weight reduction, quitting smoking, and exercise is the use of blood pressure-lowering medications.

Lisinopril can be taken by a patient without meals.

Before using Lisinopril, all patients should make sure they are properly hydrated by drinking lots of water.

Anyone experiencing swelling in their face, neck, or lips should go to the emergency room right once.

Patients who are planning a pregnancy should avoid using Lisinopril. You are advised not to use this medicine after conception as well.

Lisinopril will make you feel dizzy, so before getting up from a sitting posture, be sure you can balance yourself.

If this dizziness does not subside soon, you should consult a doctor.

Make sure your doctor always keeps an eye on your kidney, liver, and potassium levels.

Patients should avoid taking salt and potassium supplements while taking Lisinopril unless their doctor specifically instructs them to.

If you have high blood pressure, make sure to keep taking the medicine; you could feel better because high blood pressure does not usually present symptoms and indicators.

You must take this medication as prescribed by your doctor. Respect this directive to the letter.

Patients with diabetes require constant monitoring of their blood sugar levels, particularly in the initial weeks of using Lisinopril.

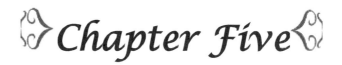

Chapter Five

Adverse Reactions in Lisinopril

Lisinopril side effects exist at various stages of development. These negative side effects are reactions to taking this drug; however some of them may quickly go away after you stop using Lisinopril.

Frequent adverse reaction

Infrequent adverse reaction

Very frequent adverse reaction

Very Frequent Adverse Reaction

- A decline in urine's capacity to concentrate.

- Lightheadedness, dizziness, or fainting upon abruptly rising from a laying or seated posture.
- Sweating.
- Cloudy vision.
- Cloudy urination.
- Confusion.
- Unusual weakness or fatigue.

Infrequent Adverse Reaction

- A common cold.
- Cough.
- Diarrhea.
- Trouble breathing
- Clogged ears.
- Stomach or abdominal discomfort
- Muscle soreness.
- Chest ache.
- Chills.
- Fever.
- Headache.
- Vocal impairment.

- Nasal obstruction
- Nausea.
- A stuffy nose.
- Sneezing.
- A throat ache.
- Vomiting.
- Appetite loss.
- Muscle soreness and aches.
- Shivering.
- Sleep issues.
- Jaw, back, and arm aches.
- Pain, tightness, and heaviness in the chest.
- An erratic and rapid heartbeat.
- A general unwell and uncomfortable sensation.
- Joint ache.

Frequent Adverse Reaction

- A diminished desire for sexual activity.
- A decreased capacity to achieve or maintain an erection.
- A decline in strength

- Sensations of burning, creeping, itching, numbness, prickling, and tingling.
- A decline in sexual prowess, passion, motivation, or performance.
- Rash.
- A whirling sensation.
- Heartburn.
- Indigestion.
- Leg cramps.
- Discomfort or distress in the stomach.
- Swelling.
- A sour or acidic stomach.
- Belching.
- A sense that you are always moving about.

Lisinopril Doses

Different strengths of Lisinopril, such as 2.5 mg, 5 mg, 10 mg, 20 mg, 30 mg, and 40 mg, are manufactured. Lisinopril doses are as follows:

Adults Suffering From Hypertension: The Initial Dosage is 10 mg once daily. The highest dosage for continuation is 80mg given once in a day, while the suggested dosage for maintenance is 20mg–40mg taken orally once daily.

Pediatrics: The lowest starting dosage required for pediatric patients is 0.07 mg once day, while the greatest initial dosage required is 5 mg once daily.

Within a week, this dose schedule may be adjusted based on the patient's blood pressure response.

If Lisinopril alone is ineffective, a lower dose of a diuretic drug may be used with it.

Adults Suffering From Heart Attacks: The starting dosage is 2.5 mg to 5 mg taken once daily. The suggested dose for maintenance should be increased as needed, and the maximum dosage for continuity is 40mg administered once day.

Take 5 mg of Lisinopril, then take 5 mg again in 24 hours. At 48 hours, double the dose. Keep taking 10 mg once each day.

Children: For dosing instructions, see your doctor.

Doses for myocardial infarction: Adults with myocardial infarction should take 5 mg once daily as their initial dose, followed by 5 mg given orally 24 hours later, and 10 mg starting 48 hours later. The suggested dosage for maintenance is 10mg taken orally once per day.

Note: Patients with lower systolic blood pressure should get 2.5 mg as their starting dosage.

Dosages for Adults with diabetic nephropathy: patient should start with a dose of 10 mg to 20 mg once daily. The highest dosage for continuation is 40mg given once day, while the suggested dosage for maintenance is 20mg-40mg taken orally once daily.

Lisinopril Warnings Regarding Missed Doses

Patients taking Lisinopril to treat hypertension may forget or miss a dosage. If you skip a dosage, it's not a crime.

If you can, take the missing dose as soon as you recall. However, if you remember that you missed a dose only a few hours before the time for the following dose, omit the missed dose and carry on with the regular dosing schedule.

Risks Associated With Lisinopril Overdose

It's possible that you accidentally overdosed on Lisinopril or did so unintentionally since you needed it to function fast or successfully. If you think you may have taken an excessive amount of this drug, get medical attention right away or dial the poison aid line right away, especially if the harm is severe.

You may reach poison control in America by dialing 1-800-222-1222.

Lisinopril Use in Pregnant and Breastfeeding Women

Lisinopril is not a drug that is recommended for use during pregnancy since it can seriously harm the fetus or even kill it.

It is strongly advised against using this drug when pregnant, especially in the second and third trimesters, since it might injure or kill the unborn child by interfering with the circulatory system.

Additionally, nursing mothers are not allowed to use Lisinopril since there is insufficient evidence to determine if the medication passes into breast milk or whether it could affect a baby who is being breastfed. Therefore, stop breastfeeding your child while using Lisinopril.

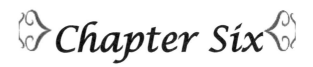

Chapter Six

Where to Buy Genuine Lisinopril Online Lawfully

Since Lisinopril needs to be prescribed by a doctor, it cannot be acquired over-the-counter.

Due to the prevalence of online pharmacies offering fake Lisinopril pills, it is important to exercise caution when choosing which ones you choose. Check to see whether the name of the online pharmacy is on the list of accredited pharmacies for Verified Internet Pharmacy Practice Site.

Verify this with the National Association of Board Pharmacy website:

There are four dosages of Lisinopril: 2.25mg, 5mg, 10mg, and 20mg.

To get your Lisinopril Tablet easily from the producing firm, CRESCENT PHARMA LIMITED, strictly follow the test below:

- Open the search tab of your preferred network browser, such as Google Chrome, UC Browser, Opera, or Internet Explorer, and type https://www.crescentpharma.com/.
- Press the system's enter key.
- It will display the CRESCENT PHARMA LIMITED homepage.
- Insert Lisinopril into the search text box and press the Enter key.
- The product will be shown, but you cannot purchase Lisinopril until you create an account with Crescent Pharma LTD.
- You can submit your demand once you have created a Crescent Account.

Alternatively

If you copy and paste the product address information below into the homepage website tab and press Enter, the product will be shown right away.

https://www.crescentpharma.com/product/lisinopril2-tablets-5mg/.

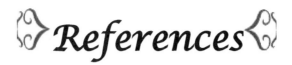

References

Bremner AD, Baur M, Oddou-Stock P, Bodin F. Valsartan: long-term efficacy and tolerability compared to Lisinopril in elderly patients with essential hypertension.Clin Exp Hypertens. 1997; 19:1263–1285. doi: 10.3109/10641969709083217.

Chavan V, Phasate P (2015) Development and validation of a UV spectrophotometric method for the determination of Lisinopril both in bulk and marketed dosage formulations. Int J Pharm Sci Res (IJPSR) 6: 394-397.

Merck Research Laboratories (2001) The Merck Index, 13th Edn., Merck & Co., White House Station, NJ, USA, pp: 989 & 86.

Mosterd A, Hoes AW, de Bruyne MC, Deckers JW, Linker DT, Hofman A, et al. Prevalence of heart failure and left ventricular dysfunction in the general population; The Rotterdam Study. Eur Heart J 1999;20:447-55.

Owan TE, Hodge DO, Herges RM, Jacobsen SJ, Roger VL, Redfield MM. Trends in prevalence and outcome of heart failure with preserved ejection fraction. N Engl J Med 2006;355:251-9.

Sharma HL, Sharma KK. Principles of pharmacology, 2nd Edn, Paras's medical publishers, Delhi, (2012) pp: 255 & 284.

Sultana N, Arayne MS, Siddiqui R, Naveed S (2012) RP-HPLC Method for the Simultaneous Determination of Lisinopril and NSAIDs in API, Pharmaceutical Formulations and Human Serum. American Journal of Analytical Chemistry 3:147-152.

The Ontarget Investigators. Telmisartan, ramipril, or both in patients at high risk for vascular events.N Engl J Med. 2008; 358:1547–1559. doi: 10.1056/NEJMoa0801317.

Wajiha Gull, Zarnab Augustine, Sidra khan, Kiran Saeed and Hira Raees. Methods of Analysis of Lisinopril: A Review. Journal of Bioequivalence & Bioavailability. Volume 9(1): 331-335 (2017) – 331.

Made in United States
Troutdale, OR
10/22/2024

24052435R00037